# Thyroidectomy Diet

## A Beginner's 2-Week Step-by-Step Guide After Thyroid Gland Removal, With Sample Recipes and a Meal Plan

mf

copyright © 2022 Brandon Gilta

All rights reserved No part of this book may be reproduced, or stored in a retrieval system, or transmitted in any form or by any means, electronic, mechanical, photocopying, recording, or otherwise, without express written permission of the publisher.

# Disclaimer

By reading this disclaimer, you are accepting the terms of the disclaimer in full. If you disagree with this disclaimer, please do not read the guide.

All of the content within this guide is provided for informational and educational purposes only, and should not be accepted as independent medical or other professional advice. The author is not a doctor, physician, nurse, mental health provider, or registered nutritionist/dietician. Therefore, using and reading this guide does not establish any form of a physician-patient relationship.

Always consult with a physician or another qualified health provider with any issues or questions you might have regarding any sort of medical condition. Do not ever disregard any qualified professional medical advice or delay seeking that advice because of anything you have read in this guide. The information in this guide is not intended to be any sort of medical advice and should not be used in lieu of any medical advice by a licensed and qualified medical professional.

The information in this guide has been compiled from a variety of known sources. However, the author cannot attest to or guarantee the accuracy of each source and thus should not be held liable for any errors or omissions.

You acknowledge that the publisher of this guide will not be held liable for any loss or damage of any kind incurred as a result of this guide or the reliance on any information provided within this guide. You acknowledge and agree that you assume all risk and responsibility for any action you undertake in response to the information in this guide.

Using this guide does not guarantee any particular result (e.g., weight loss or a cure). By reading this guide, you acknowledge that there are no guarantees to any specific outcome or results you can expect.

All product names, diet plans, or names used in this guide are for identification purposes only and are the property of their respective owners. The use of these names does not imply endorsement. All other trademarks cited herein are the property of their respective owners.

Where applicable, this guide is not intended to be a substitute for the original work of this diet plan and is, at most, a supplement to the original work for this diet plan and never a direct substitute. This guide is a personal expression of the facts of that diet plan.

Where applicable, persons shown in the cover images are stock photography models and the publisher has obtained the rights to use the images through license agreements with third-party stock image companies.

# Table of Contents

**Introduction**     7
**What Is Thyroid Disease?**     10
    Symptoms of Thyroid Diseases     10
    Causes of Thyroid Diseases     12
    Diseases Related to Hypothyroidism     14
    Diseases Related to Hyperthyroidism     16
    Lifestyle Changes to Manage Thyroid Disease     16
**What Is Thyroidectomy?**     20
    The Surgical Process     20
    Types of Thyroidectomy Procedures     22
    Subtotal Thyroidectomy     23
**Preparing for Thyroidectomy: Steps to Take Before Surgery**     26
    Personal Care and Restrictions     26
    Day of Surgery: What to Do     27
    Post-thyroidectomy: Recovery and Expectations     28
**Post-Thyroidectomy Diet**     30
    Principles of the Post-thyroidectomy Diet     30
    Benefits of the Post-thyroidectomy Diet     32
    Disadvantages of Post-Thyroidectomy Diet     33
**A Step-by-Step Guide To Get Started With the Post-Thyroidectomy Diet**     35
    Step 1: Consult with Your Nutrition Specialist     35
    Step 2: Embrace Nutrient Diversity in Your Meals     37
    Step 3: Monitor Calcium and Vitamin D Intake     38
    Step 4: Stay Hydrated and Minimize Caffeine     39
    Step 5: Adjust Fiber Intake According to Digestive Comfort     40
    Foods to Eat     41
    Foods to Avoid     43
    Food list to consume after thyroidectomy     45

| | |
|---|---|
| **Diet Plan Implementation** | **47** |
| Week 1: Types of Food | 47 |
| Important tips to relax your throat while eating | 49 |
| Week 2: 7-day Meal Plan | 50 |
| **Sample Recipes** | **52** |
| Asian-Style Vegetable Soup | 53 |
| Lentil Soup | 55 |
| Meaty Cauliflower Soup | 57 |
| Tomato and Basil Soup | 58 |
| Sweet Potato Soup | 59 |
| Minestrone Soup | 60 |
| Broccoli Soup with Tumeric and Ginger | 62 |
| Vegetable Stew | 63 |
| Garlic Hummus | 65 |
| Salmon and Asparagus | 66 |
| Tahini Salmon | 67 |
| Chicken Breast Delight | 69 |
| Steak with Olive Oil | 70 |
| Garlic Broccoli Salad | 72 |
| Spinach and Watercress Salad | 73 |
| Vegetable Broth | 74 |
| Fruit and Dark Greens Salad | 76 |
| **Conclusion** | **78** |
| **FAQ** | **81** |
| **References and Helpful Links** | **84** |

# Introduction

Understanding the thyroidectomy process is crucial, and this guide is meticulously crafted to act as your reliable companion throughout this transformative journey. It's a pivotal moment when you decide to undergo surgery, and being armed with knowledge not only empowers you but also quells the swirling tides of apprehension.

Your thyroid, that butterfly-shaped gland sitting discreetly at the base of your neck, plays a pivotal role in regulating countless bodily functions. When this gland begins to act up, whether due to cancer, benign nodules, a goiter, or an overactive thyroid condition, it can throw your whole system off balance. It's at this intersection of necessity and health that a thyroidectomy procedure becomes not just a medical term but a personal milestone.

Why are you walking down this path, and how do you prepare for what's to come? These questions might hover in your mind as you embark on this journey. Whether it's a nagging concern over potential risks or simply curiosity about the recovery process, gathering knowledge empowers you to approach your thyroidectomy with confidence.

In this guide, we will talk about the following;

- Thyroidectomy: Procedure and Types
- What is Thyroidectomy? Types of Thyroidectomy Procedures
- Symptoms and Causes of Thyroid Diseases
- Diseases Related to Hypothyroidism and Hyperthyroidism
- Preparing for Thyroidectomy: Steps to Take Before Surgery
- Post-thyroidectomy Diet
- Principles, Benefits, and Disadvantages of Post-thyroidectomy Diet
- Foods to Eat and to Avoid
- Sample Meal Plan and Recipes

Instead of walking into the unknown, equip yourself with clarity about what your thyroidectomy will entail. Knowledge is both comfort and power when facing a medical procedure. Consider the reassurance of having a comprehensive guide at your disposal that navigates you through the pre-surgery planning, accompanies you with thorough guidance during the operation, and offers unwavering support as you recuperate. You won't just be another patient in the lineup; you'll be at the center of a compassionate team whose goal is to enhance your healing and restore your balance.

As the pages of this guide unfold, we invite you to dive deeper into the world of thyroidectomy. Learn about the different types of procedures, what you can expect before, during, and after surgery, and how to manage recovery with grace. You've taken the first, most crucial step by seeking understanding, and we're here to illuminate the rest of your path.

Embarking on this procedure is undoubtedly a significant decision, one that comes with many questions and considerations. But you're not alone. By the end of this guide, you'll have a comprehensive understanding of what thyroidectomy entails, equipping you with the knowledge to face the upcoming procedure with clarity and calm. So let's begin this journey together, shall we?

# What Is Thyroid Disease?

Thyroid disease is a term that refers to the malfunctioning of the thyroid gland, which is responsible for producing hormones that regulate the body's metabolism. Disorders can result in the production of either too much or too little hormone, affecting overall health and bodily functions. Treatment approaches vary and may include medication, radioiodine therapy, or surgery, depending on the specific condition.

Diagnosis is typically achieved through clinical evaluation and specialized blood tests that assess thyroid hormone levels. Proper management of thyroid disease is critical to maintaining metabolic balance and ensuring overall well-being.

## Symptoms of Thyroid Diseases

Thyroid disease symptoms can vary widely depending on whether the thyroid is overactive (hyperthyroidism) or underactive (hypothyroidism). Here are some common symptoms for both conditions:

**Hyperthyroidism Symptoms**

- Unexpected weight loss, even when appetite and food consumption remain normal or increase
- Rapid heartbeat (tachycardia), palpitations, or irregular heartbeat (arrhythmias)
- Nervousness, anxiety, and irritability
- Tremors in the hands and fingers
- Sweating and sensitivity to heat
- Changes in menstrual patterns
- More frequent bowel movements
- Enlarged thyroid gland (goiter)
- Exhaustion and lack of muscular strength.
- Difficulty sleeping (insomnia)

**Hypothyroidism Symptoms**

- Fatigue and sluggishness
- Unexplained weight gain
- Increased sensitivity to cold
- Constipation
- Dry skin
- Puffy face
- Hoarseness
- Diminished muscle strength.
- Increased levels of cholesterol in the blood.
- Discomfort, sensitivity, and rigidity in muscles.
- Discomfort, rigidity, or inflammation in your articulations.

- Menstrual cycles that are more intense than usual or inconsistent.
- Thinning hair
- Slowed heart rate
- Depression
- Impaired memory

Symptoms of thyroid disease can be subtle or develop slowly over time, making them easy to overlook. If you experience any persistent symptoms, it is important to seek medical attention for proper diagnosis and treatment.

## Causes of Thyroid Diseases

Thyroid diseases can be caused by a variety of factors, including:

### Autoimmune Disorders

Conditions such as Hashimoto's thyroiditis and Graves' disease occur when the immune system mistakenly attacks the thyroid gland, leading to hypothyroidism or hyperthyroidism, respectively.

### Iodine Imbalance

Too much or too little iodine in the diet can cause thyroid dysfunction since iodine is critical for the production of thyroid hormones.

## Genetic Predisposition

There is often a hereditary component to thyroid disorders, making individuals with a family history of thyroid diseases more susceptible.

## Thyroid Nodules

The presence of nodules or lumps within the thyroid gland can affect its function, sometimes causing overproduction or underproduction of hormones.

## Inflammation

Thyroiditis, an inflammation of the thyroid, which can be due to an autoimmune reaction or other causes, can lead to temporary hyperthyroidism or a longer-term hypothyroid condition.

## Pituitary Gland Malfunctions

Since the pituitary gland regulates thyroid hormone production, any disorder affecting this master gland can also influence thyroid function.

## Thyroid Cancer

Thyroid cancer can alter the normal functioning of the thyroid gland, though it might not always cause overt symptoms.

**Pregnancy**

Some women develop thyroid problems during or after pregnancy due to the complex hormonal changes occurring during this time.

**Radiation Exposure**

Exposure to radiation, especially in the head and neck area, can increase the risk of thyroid disease.

**Certain Medications**

Some medications, like lithium, can impact thyroid hormone production.

Understanding the specific cause of a thyroid disorder is crucial for proper treatment and management of the condition.

## Diseases Related to Hypothyroidism

**Thyroiditis Thyroiditis**

This involves the swelling or irritation of the thyroid gland, leading to excess or inadequate production of thyroid hormones. It progresses through three phases:

- Thyrotoxic Phase: Excessive hormone production due to inflammation.
- Hypothyroid Phase: Reduced hormone secretion following prolonged excess.

- Euthyroid Phase: Temporary normalization of hormone levels during recovery. Causes include antibodies, viruses, bacteria, and radiation, with antibodies being the most common initiator. Infections and medication side effects can also contribute. Diagnostic tests include thyroid function and antibody tests, as well as ultrasound. Symptoms vary based on the phases and may include fatigue, constipation, depression, rapid heart rate, weight loss, anxiety, and tremors.

## Hashimoto's Thyroiditis

This autoimmune condition results in the immune system attacking the thyroid gland, leading to symptoms such as fatigue, feeling cold, depression, hair loss, and slow heartbeat. Diagnosis involves tests like Thyroid-stimulating hormone and antithyroid antibody tests, as well as Free T4 test.

## Postpartum Thyroiditis

Occurring after childbirth, this temporary condition affects around 5% of pregnant women and is caused by antithyroid antibodies. Symptoms, appearing 1 to 6 months post-childbirth, may include rapid heart rate, weight loss, increased body temperature, and hair loss.

# Diseases Related to Hyperthyroidism

### Graves' Disease

Characterized by an overactive thyroid, Graves' disease predominantly affects women aged 30 to 50, especially those with a family history of thyroid disease. The cause is not fully understood, but it's believed that something in the body triggers the excessive production of thyroid-stimulating immunoglobulin (TSI), leading to symptoms such as goiter, heat intolerance, eye inflammation, and fatigue. Diagnosis involves blood tests, Radioactive iodine uptake (RAIU), and Thyroid scans.

### Thyroid Nodule

Thyroid nodules are abnormal lumps of thyroid cells that can lead to cancer in less than 5% of cases. Causes are uncertain, but risk factors include family history and iodine deficiency. Types of nodules include colloid nodules, thyroid cysts, inflammatory nodules, and thyroid cancer.

Symptoms encompass irritability, hoarseness, enlarged thyroid gland, changes in appetite, skin flushing, and depression. Diagnostic tests include a thyroid scan, ultrasound, and fine needle biopsy of the thyroid gland.

## Lifestyle Changes to Manage Thyroid Disease

Managing thyroid disease often includes a combination of medical treatment and lifestyle adjustments. Here are some general lifestyle changes that can help manage thyroid conditions:

**Healthy Diet**

Eating a well-balanced diet that's high in fruits, vegetables, and lean proteins can support overall health. Certain nutrients like iodine, selenium, and zinc are important for thyroid function, but it's essential to consult a healthcare provider before making any significant changes or starting supplements.

**Regular Exercise**

Engaging in regular physical activity helps with weight management, mood improvement, and energy levels, which can be affected by thyroid disorders.

**Stress Management**

Chronic stress can negatively impact thyroid function. Techniques like meditation, deep breathing exercises, yoga, or other relaxation practices can be beneficial.

**Adequate Sleep**

Sufficient rest is crucial for the body to repair itself and regulate hormones effectively. Aim for 7-9 hours of quality sleep per night.

**Avoiding Certain Foods**

Some foods, like soy and cruciferous vegetables, may affect thyroid function, especially in individuals with iodine deficiency. It's important to discuss dietary concerns with a healthcare provider.

**Limiting Goitrogens**

These substances, found in certain foods like cabbage, broccoli, and kale, can interfere with thyroid hormone production. Cooking these foods can minimize their goitrogenic effect.

**Avoiding Excessive Intake of Raw Iodine**

While iodine is vital for thyroid health, too much of it can be harmful, especially in certain types of thyroid disease.

**Quitting Smoking**

The toxins in cigarettes can affect the thyroid gland, especially in people with an existing thyroid condition.

**Monitoring Thyroid Function**

Regularly check your thyroid hormone levels as advised by your healthcare professional to adjust lifestyle habits and medication as needed.

**Patient Education**

Understanding the condition can promote better management, including recognizing symptoms that indicate the need for treatment adjustment.

**Medication Compliance**

If you're prescribed thyroid hormone replacement or other medications, take them as directed and consult with your doctor about any side effects.

With proper management, individuals with thyroid disease can live a healthy and fulfilling life. However, it's essential to remember that each person's experience with thyroid disease is unique, and treatment may need to be adjusted accordingly.

# What Is Thyroidectomy?

Thyroidectomy is a medical operation that involves the surgical removal of the entire thyroid gland (total thyroidectomy) or a portion of it (partial thyroidectomy). The procedure is indicated for several thyroid-related conditions such as cancer, noncancerous enlargement of the thyroid (goiter), overactive thyroid (hyperthyroidism), and suspicious nodules.

The extent of removal depends on the reason for the surgery. Conducted under general anesthesia, a thyroidectomy can help manage symptoms and prevent further complications associated with thyroid disease.

## The Surgical Process

Thyroid surgeries are conducted in a hospital setting. Patients are required to fast, and refrain from food or drink, starting from midnight before the day of surgery.

Upon arriving at the hospital, patients go through the admission process and are directed to the pre-operative area. There, patients change into a hospital gown, and an intravenous (IV) line is inserted into the wrist or arm to administer fluids and medication.

Patients will have a pre-surgical consultation with their surgeon to review the procedure, undergo a brief physical examination, and have any lingering questions addressed. An anesthesiologist will also discuss the administration of anesthesia to ensure comfort throughout the surgery.

When it's time for the surgery, patients are taken to the operating room where the anesthesia is delivered through the IV. Although the medication may initially cause a cold or tingling sensation, it quickly induces deep sleep.

During the procedure, the surgeon makes an incision on the neck to expose the thyroid gland. Depending on the condition being treated, either a portion or the entirety of the gland is removed. Given the intricate anatomy surrounding the thyroid, including important nerves and glands, the surgery may last two hours.

Post-surgery, patients awaken in the recovery room, where medical staff closely monitor comfort levels, and vital signs, and administer pain relief as necessary. Once stable, patients are moved to a standard hospital room for further observation, which typically lasts between 24 to 48 hours.

## Types of Thyroidectomy Procedures

Thyroidectomy procedures vary depending on the extent and nature of the thyroid issue. Below are the primary types of thyroidectomies:

**Thyroid Lobectomy**

A thyroid lobectomy, also called a hemithyroidectomy, is a surgical procedure to treat thyroid conditions by removing one of the two lobes. It is used when the issue is limited to one part of the gland, preserving the remaining thyroid tissue and function.

Conditions requiring a lobectomy include non-cancerous nodules, follicular neoplasms, unilateral Graves' disease, and early-stage cancers within one lobe. During the operation, surgeons carefully remove the affected lobe while preserving critical structures like the parathyroid glands and laryngeal nerves.

This prevents complications such as voice changes or hoarseness. The procedure also allows for the evaluation of nearby lymph nodes for cancer spread. A lobectomy is typically recommended for lesions up to 4 cm in size, based on balancing effective treatment and minimizing complications.

After the procedure, some patients may need thyroid hormone supplementation depending on the function of the remaining thyroid tissue. In summary, a thyroid lobectomy is a focused alternative to total thyroidectomy, effectively treating localized thyroid diseases while preserving gland function and minimizing complications.

## Subtotal Thyroidectomy

A subtotal thyroidectomy, also known as a near-total thyroidectomy, involves surgically removing the majority of the thyroid gland while leaving a small segment of tissue. This procedure aims to eliminate problematic thyroid tissue responsible for diseases while preserving some hormone-producing capabilities.

Conditions that may require a subtotal thyroidectomy include Graves' disease, toxic multinodular goiter, and large or symptomatic non-toxic goiters. In some cases, patients with small thyroid cancers may also be considered for this surgery.

The decision to perform a subtotal thyroidectomy instead of a total thyroidectomy is influenced by the potential to maintain natural thyroid function and avoid lifelong dependency on hormone replacement medications. The remaining thyroid tissue is expected to produce enough hormones to meet the body's needs.

However, outcomes can vary, and some patients may experience hypothyroidism due to inadequate hormone production by the remaining tissue. Regular monitoring of thyroid-stimulating hormone levels is necessary, and hormone replacement therapy may be required.

Subtotal thyroidectomy aims to address thyroid-related diseases while preserving part of the thyroid's function. However, close postoperative monitoring and potential hormone replacement therapy are necessary to manage hypothyroidism.

**Total Thyroidectomy**

A total thyroidectomy is a surgical procedure that involves complete removal of the thyroid gland. This approach is often recommended for advanced-stage thyroid cancer or when there is a high risk of recurrence or metastasis. The removal of the gland ensures excision of potentially malignant tissue, which is crucial for prognosis and long-term survival.

Besides cancer treatment, a total thyroidectomy may be performed for conditions like large goiters, which can cause compressive symptoms. It is also an option for hyperthyroidism unresponsive to other treatments or caused by Graves' disease. The surgery addresses the overproduction of thyroid hormone.

Factors like glandular size, extent of enlargement, nodules, inflammation, and potential malignancy are considered before deciding on a total thyroidectomy. A comprehensive diagnostic workup, including imaging and possibly biopsy, guides the surgical plan.

After the surgery, patients will experience loss of natural thyroid function, necessitating lifelong hormone replacement therapy. Levothyroxine, a synthetic form of thyroid hormone, is prescribed to maintain normal metabolic rates, body temperature, and energy levels.

It is important to note the risks associated with a total thyroidectomy, including damage to nerves resulting in voice changes, injury to parathyroid glands causing hypocalcemia, and general risks of infection or bleeding. Specialized surgeons experienced in thyroid operations minimize these risks.

Patients who undergo a total thyroidectomy require long-term follow-up to monitor hormone levels and adjust medication dosage. Regular blood tests ensure effective replacement therapy.

A total thyroidectomy is a definitive surgical intervention for various thyroid conditions, especially thyroid cancer. It offers a high chance of remission or cure but requires lifelong hormone replacement therapy and ongoing medical monitoring for optimal health outcomes.

# Preparing for Thyroidectomy: Steps to Take Before Surgery

If you're scheduled for a thyroidectomy, it's essential to prepare both physically and logistically. Here's a structured guide on how to get ready:

## Personal Care and Restrictions

- Bathe the evening before a morning surgery, or in the morning if your surgery is later in the day, to reduce the risk of infection.
- Abstain from eating at least 12 hours before your procedure to avoid complications during anesthesia.
- Refrain from alcohol consumption for a full 24 hours before the surgery.
- If you smoke, it's critical to quit smoking at least four weeks before your operation to decrease the likelihood of postoperative complications.

## Valuables and Personal Items

Leave valuables such as cash and jewelry at home to prevent loss for which the hospital cannot be held accountable.

## Medication Management

Consult with your doctor about any medications you're taking. Blood thinners like aspirin, ibuprofen, and certain herbal or vitamin supplements may need to be discontinued a week before surgery due to their potential effect on bleeding risks and anesthesia.

## Anesthesia Consultation

Have a discussion with an anesthesiologist about your anesthesia options. This might involve an in-depth conversation over the phone or an in-person meeting to review the associated risks and benefits.

## Diagnostic Procedures

Undergo necessary diagnostic tests such as a thyroid ultrasound, CT scans, MRI, and blood tests. These will help your healthcare team assess the specific nature of your thyroid condition.

# Day of Surgery: What to Do

The day of your procedure will follow a carefully outlined protocol:

- ***Documentation***: Bring all essential documents, including the surgeon's orders and your ID card.

- *Check-In Process*: Upon arrival, you'll be asked to verify your identity and share your medical record, and the surgical site will be marked for precision.
- *Anesthesia Administration*: Anesthesia will be provided to ensure you are comfortable and pain-free during the surgery. This could range from general anesthesia to localized options for the targeted area.
- *Hyperthyroidism Management*: If you've been diagnosed with hyperthyroidism, you may receive medication to manage your hormone levels before the surgery begins.
- *Post-Surgery Transport*: Arrange for a companion who can drive you home safely after the operation.

## Post-thyroidectomy: Recovery and Expectations

After your thyroidectomy, here's what you can generally expect:

- *Physical Sensations*: It's normal to experience some throat soreness, neck discomfort, difficulty swallowing, or changes in your voice temporarily following the procedure.
- *Dietary Considerations*: Food intake may be limited on the night of your surgery, but most patients resume their regular diet by the next day.

- ***Scarring and Healing***: A horizontal incision resulting in a 3 to 4-inch scar near your collar line is typical. Although noticeable initially, the scar should blend into the natural folds of your neck skin and become less prominent over time.
- ***Fatigue Management***: Feeling tired is a common postoperative symptom, stemming from the body channeling energy into healing and the adjustment of metabolism due to altered thyroid hormone production. Whether partially or fully removed, the change in your thyroid's function can affect your metabolic rate and energy levels.
- ***Calcium Monitoring***: The surgery can affect parathyroid glands, potentially causing a dip in calcium levels. Be aware of symptoms like tingling or numbness in your lips or fingers, indicative of this change.

By understanding the before and after steps of a thyroidectomy, you can better prepare for a smooth surgery and recovery process. If you have any concerns or need further clarification, always consult with your healthcare provider for personalized advice.

# Post-Thyroidectomy Diet

After a thyroidectomy, patients are often required to follow a specific dict tailored to support their recovery and adjust to the changes in their body's hormone regulation. The Post-thyroidectomy Diet focuses on nourishing the body with foods that aid in healing, maintain energy levels, and contribute to overall well-being during this critical period.

Given that the thyroid plays a key role in metabolism, dietary adjustments may also help manage weight and provide the right balance of nutrients. This diet is designed to work alongside prescribed medications and therapies, facilitating a smoother transition back to daily activities while monitoring and supporting thyroid hormone levels post-surgery.

## Principles of the Post-thyroidectomy Diet

The basic principles of the Post-thyroidectomy Diet revolve around supporting healing, maintaining balanced nutrient intake, and accommodating the body's adjusted metabolic needs. Here are several foundational guidelines:

- *Adequate hydration*: Prioritize fluid intake to stay hydrated, which is crucial for healing and overall health.
- *Protein-rich foods*: Include a sufficient amount of protein to aid in tissue repair and recovery.
- *Calcium and vitamin D*: Focus on calcium and vitamin D to support bone health, especially since thyroid surgery can affect calcium levels.
- *Fiber intake*: Consume fiber-rich foods to maintain digestive health and prevent constipation, which can be a post-operative concern.
- *Controlled iodine levels*: If required, manage iodine intake as it can influence thyroid hormone production, particularly if you're on replacement therapy.
- *Balanced meals*: Ensure meals are well-balanced with vegetables, fruits, whole grains, and lean proteins to aid in overall wellness.
- *Limit goitrogenic foods*: Some may need to moderate consumption of goitrogens, substances that can interfere with thyroid function, depending on their physician's advice.
- *Moderate portions*: Monitor portion sizes to help regulate weight since metabolism may fluctuate after thyroid removal.
- *Avoid processed foods*: Minimize intake of processed foods, which can be high in unhelpful nutrients like sugars, fats, and salts.

- *Regular monitoring*: Keep track of how your body responds to different foods and maintain regular communication with a dietitian or healthcare provider for personalized adjustments.

Remember, individual dietary needs can vary greatly, so these principles should be tailored to each patient's specific circumstances, often with the guidance of a healthcare professional.

## Benefits of the Post-thyroidectomy Diet

When considering the post-thyroidectomy diet, it's essential to understand the potential benefits. Proper nutrition can promote quicker recovery and better overall health after thyroid surgery. A well-planned diet can:

- *Improved Wound Healing*: A post-thyroidectomy diet rich in protein and essential nutrients, like vitamin C and zinc, can help the body's tissue repair process and promote better wound healing after surgery.
- *Stabilized Metabolic Function*: Because the thyroid gland plays a pivotal role in metabolism, adjusting your diet to include balanced portions of carbohydrates, fats, and proteins can help stabilize metabolic functions post-surgery.
- *Weight Management Support*: The diet helps manage weight fluctuations by providing guidance on appropriate caloric intake and nutritious food choices

to compensate for potential changes in metabolism following thyroid removal.
- *Adequate Calcium and Vitamin D Intake*: Thyroidectomy may affect calcium levels due to potential impacts on parathyroid glands; including calcium and vitamin D in the diet is key to maintaining bone health.
- *Reduced Gastrointestinal Discomfort*: A diet tailored to be easily digestible with adequate fiber can alleviate common post-operative digestive issues, ensuring comfort and promoting gut health as the body heals.

By considering these benefits and tailoring the diet to one's specific needs, patients can promote a smoother recovery and improve their overall health post-thyroidectomy.

## Disadvantages of Post-Thyroidectomy Diet

Although a post-thyroidectomy diet has numerous benefits, there are a few disadvantages to be aware of as well. These may include:

- *Dietary Restrictions*: Post-thyroidectomy, individuals may need to adhere to certain dietary restrictions which can limit food choices and make meal planning more challenging.
- *Nutrient Deficiency Risks*: Without proper planning, the diet could lead to deficiencies in crucial nutrients that were previously regulated by a healthy thyroid.

- ***Social and Lifestyle Adjustments***: Following a specialized diet may require significant lifestyle changes that impact social activities and dining experiences.
- ***Short-Term Digestive Adjustments***: Initially, the body might experience digestive issues as it adapts to new dietary changes, which can be inconvenient and uncomfortable.
- ***Maintenance of Calcium and Vitamin D Levels***: Ensuring adequate levels of calcium and vitamin D can be demanding, requiring consistent monitoring and potential supplementation.

Despite these disadvantages, the benefits of following a Post-thyroidectomy diet often outweigh these challenges, particularly in terms of promoting recovery, maintaining balanced energy levels, and supporting overall health after thyroid surgery. With careful planning and possible consultation with a healthcare provider or dietitian, these disadvantages can be managed effectively.

# A Step-by-Step Guide To Get Started With the Post-Thyroidectomy Diet

Recovering from thyroidectomy requires not just rest, but also a nourishing diet that caters to your new health needs. Here's a step-by-step guide to help you navigate your post-surgery nutrition effectively.

## Step 1: Consult with Your Nutrition Specialist

Begin your post-thyroidectomy journey by scheduling a detailed consultation with a qualified dietitian or nutritionist specializing in endocrine health and post-surgical recovery. Partnering with an expert who understands the intricacies of thyroid health and the changes your body will experience post-surgery is crucial.

During the initial session, expect a comprehensive evaluation of your current health, diet, and any specific symptoms or challenges you may face after thyroidectomy. Your nutrition specialist will use this information to create a customized diet plan that supports your body's unique needs during the healing process.

Thyroid-related treatments can impact nutrient absorption and metabolism, so your specialist will emphasize the importance of specific vitamins and minerals for recovery. They will explain how these nutrients contribute to tissue repair, inflammation reduction, and overall well-being.

Bone health and cellular function rely on minerals like calcium and phosphorus, which may require special attention after a thyroidectomy. Your nutritional consultant will monitor your blood levels of these minerals and provide supplementation recommendations or a curated list of foods to maintain balance.

In addition to nutrient focus, your nutritionist will guide you on general eating patterns that promote healing, including meal timing, portion sizes, and structuring meals and snacks for sustained energy and metabolism.

This consultative process aims to empower you with knowledge and strategies for long-term health. Understanding how food affects your body after thyroidectomy and making necessary adjustments ensures a smoother recovery and a healthier future.

Open communication with your nutrition specialist is key. Ask questions, share concerns, and provide feedback for ongoing tailoring of your diet plan to align with your recovery milestones and changing nutritional needs. This step sets the foundation for nurturing your body with precision and care after thyroidectomy.

## Step 2: Embrace Nutrient Diversity in Your Meals

As you transition to the next phase of your post-surgical nutrition plan, focus on integrating a wide variety of nutrients through a diverse diet. Achieving a balance of macro and micronutrients is crucial for healing and recovery after thyroidectomy.

A balanced meal is like a symphony, with proteins, carbohydrates, and fats each playing a vital role. Proteins are essential for tissue repair and immune function during recovery. Carbohydrates provide energy and mental alertness. Fats aid in the absorption of fat-soluble vitamins and maintain cell health. Micronutrients from diverse food sources support various bodily functions, from bone health to antioxidant protection.

Plan meals around colorful vegetables, fruits, lean proteins, whole grains, and healthy fats. Each food group brings its micronutrients. For example, leafy greens and brightly colored vegetables offer antioxidants, while citrus fruits and berries provide immune support with vitamin C. Whole grains provide fiber for digestive health and blood sugar management.

Healthy fats, like those in avocados, nuts, and seeds, supply essential fatty acids with anti-inflammatory properties. By valuing nutrient diversity in meal planning, you optimize your body's natural repair mechanisms and improve overall well-being. Remember to consider individual tolerance and dietary restrictions and work closely with healthcare or nutrition professionals for ongoing guidance.

## Step 3: Monitor Calcium and Vitamin D Intake

In the third step, it's crucial to carefully manage calcium and vitamin D intake, as these nutrients are vital for recovery. The procedure can affect the parathyroid glands, which regulate calcium balance. To prevent complications, incorporate calcium-rich foods like dairy, leafy greens, and fortified options into your diet. Vitamin D, known as the "sunshine vitamin," is also important for calcium absorption and bone health.

Get enough through sources like fatty fish, egg yolks, and enriched products. Your healthcare provider may recommend supplements, but regular blood tests are essential to monitor levels and make adjustments. Be cautious with supplementation and seek professional guidance. Prioritizing these nutrients supports your post-thyroidectomy recovery and overall well-being.

## Step 4: Stay Hydrated and Minimize Caffeine

After thyroid surgery, maintaining proper hydration is crucial. Water is essential for healing, serving multiple critical functions. Aim for at least eight 8-ounce glasses of water daily to ensure optimal blood volume and pressure, facilitating nutrient circulation and tissue repair. Adequate hydration also aids in waste elimination post-operation.

Water also plays a pivotal role in maintaining energy levels. During recovery, fatigue is common, and dehydration can exacerbate this feeling of tiredness. Ensuring you're well-hydrated helps combat this issue, providing you with a more consistent energy supply throughout the day.

Although caffeine is a commonly enjoyed stimulant, it may not be as beneficial during your recovery. It has a diuretic effect, potentially leading to dehydration if not balanced with additional water intake. Furthermore, caffeine can impact calcium metabolism. Considering the importance of calcium in post-surgical care, it's wise to moderate caffeine consumption by choosing decaffeinated coffee, tea, or herbal alternatives. These options can still provide a comforting warm beverage without the negative effects of caffeine.

Herbal teas, in particular, can be a soothing and hydrating choice, with some varieties like chamomile or peppermint offering their own set of therapeutic benefits. Such herbal infusions can contribute to your fluid intake while also providing relaxation and digestive support—both welcome effects during recovery.

By prioritizing hydration and minimizing caffeine, you will be taking yet another step towards a smooth and swift recovery, ensuring that your body has the necessary resources to heal effectively while avoiding substances that could potentially impair this process. Remember to listen to your body's signals for thirst and keep water accessible throughout the day to encourage regular sipping.

## Step 5: Adjust Fiber Intake According to Digestive Comfort

Finally, pay attention to your body's signals and adjust your fiber intake accordingly. Anesthesia and pain medications can sometimes slow down your digestive system, leading to constipation. If this happens, slowly increase your intake of fiber from fruits, vegetables, and whole grains. Alternatively, if you experience loose stools, you might need to ease off high-fiber foods temporarily and focus on soothing, easy-to-digest meals like broth, yogurt, and soft-cooked eggs.

Through each of these steps, track how your body responds, and don't hesitate to seek further advice from your healthcare provider. They can make any necessary dietary tweaks and ensure that your recovery is both comfortable and hastened by your nutritional choices. Remember, a well-planned diet after thyroidectomy isn't just about healing in the short term—it's also about setting the foundation for your long-term health and well-being.

## Foods to Eat

After a thyroidectomy, it's important to focus on a diet that not only supports your overall health but also addresses specific nutritional needs due to the absence of the thyroid gland. Here's a list of foods to consider incorporating into your post-thyroidectomy diet:

**Calcium and Vitamin D Rich Foods:**
- Low-fat milk, cheese, and other dairy products
- Fortified plant-based milk (almond, soy, etc.)
- Fatty fish (salmon, mackerel, sardines)
- Fortified cereals and orange juice
- Egg yolks

**Iodine-rich Foods (if recommended by your doctor):**
- Iodized salt (in moderation)
- Seaweed varieties such as nori or kelp
- Cod and shrimp
- Dairy products
- Eggs

**Fiber-Rich Foods:**
- Whole grain bread and cereals
- Brown rice and quinoa

- Beans, lentils, and legumes
- Fresh fruits and vegetables

**Protein-Rich Foods:**

- Lean meats like chicken and turkey
- Fish and seafood
- Eggs
- Tofu and tempeh
- Nuts and seeds

**Iron-Rich Foods:**

- Red meat in moderation
- Poultry and fish
- Legumes like chickpeas and lentils
- Green leafy vegetables (spinach, kale)
- Fortified cereals

**Antioxidant-rich Foods for immune support:**

- Berries (strawberries, blueberries, raspberries)
- Dark chocolate (in moderation)
- Green tea
- Nuts (walnuts, almonds)

**Healthy Fats:**

- Avocados
- Olive oil and other plant-based oils
- Nuts and seeds

- Fatty fish

Always remember to stay hydrated by drinking plenty of water throughout the day and avoid or limit foods with high amounts of added sugars and unhealthy fats.

It is crucial to tailor your diet to your unique needs, so consult with a healthcare professional or a registered dietitian specializing in thyroid health who can create a personalized meal plan based on your requirements.

## Foods to Avoid

After a thyroidectomy, certain foods should be limited or avoided to support healing and maintain optimal health. Here are some types of foods you might consider reducing or eliminating from your diet:

### Goitrogenic Foods

Some foods can interfere with thyroid hormone production and are known as goitrogens. These are especially important to avoid or limit if you still have some remaining thyroid tissue or if you are on thyroid hormone replacement therapy. Examples include:

- Soy products (tofu, tempeh, edamame)
- Cruciferous vegetables (cabbage, broccoli, kale, cauliflower) when eaten in excessive amounts and raw
- Certain fruits like peaches, pears, and strawberries
- Foods rich in gluten if you have gluten sensitivity

## Foods High in Sugars and Refined Carbohydrates

- Sweets, candies, and chocolates
- Sugary drinks, including sodas and fruit juices
- White bread, pasta, and rice
- Pastries, cakes, and other baked goods

## Iodine Excess

- Seaweed or kelp supplements
- Iodine-fortified foods in excess (consult your doctor for appropriate iodine levels)

## High-Sodium Foods

- Processed foods like canned soups, ready meals, and deli meats
- Salty snacks
- Foods with added salt or salty seasonings

## Fatty, Fried, and Fast Foods

- Fast food items
- Fried foods and those with trans fats
- High-fat meats and dairy products

## Caffeine and Alcohol

- Coffee and tea in large amounts
- Alcoholic beverages

**Certain Supplements and Herbal Products**

Some may affect hormone levels or interact with your thyroid medication. Always consult with your healthcare provider before taking any new supplements or herbal remedies.

**Artificial Additives**

- Artificial sweeteners
- Preservatives and colorings found in many processed foods

While these are general guidelines, individual dietary needs can vary, especially after surgery. Monitoring how certain foods affect your body and working closely with a dietician or nutritionist can help you develop a personalized eating plan that supports your post-thyroidectomy health.

## Food list to consume after thyroidectomy

We have created a food list for you to try after your thyroidectomy.

- Asian-Style Vegetable Soup
- Lentil Soup
- Meaty Cauliflower Soup
- Tomato and Basil Soup
- Sweet Potato Soup
- Minestrone Soup
- Broccoli Soup with Turmeric and Ginger
- Vegetable stew

- Garlic Hummus
- Salmon and Asparagus
- Tahini Salmon
- Chicken Breast Delight
- Steak with Olive Oil
- Garlic Broccoli Salad
- Spinach and Watercress Salad
- Vegetable Broth
- Fruit and Dark Greens Salad

The recipes of these dishes are shared in the Sample Recipes chapter.

# Diet Plan Implementation

## Week 1: Types of Food

**Soft Food**

In the first week, a patient can have trouble eating normal food because of a sore throat. So, to overcome this problem, a patient must eat soft foods that can easily be swallowed.

*__The following is the list of soft foods compiled for your help:__*

- Scrambled eggs
- Ice-cream
- Smoothies
- Mild soups
- Strained vegetable soups
- Mashed potatoes
- Pasta
- Oatmeal
- Milkshakes
- Fruit Juices (Not packaged)

**Cold Foods**

Some people experience a fever after a thyroidectomy. It can be due to an irritated throat. The throat will be irritated because of inflammation after the surgery. In this case, cold foods are essential for relaxing the throat.

Some of the cold foods are listed below:

- Shakes
- Yogurt
- Smoothies
- Ice chips
- Popsicles

**Protein Foods**

Protein is essential for your body to heal following surgery. Keep in mind that it is a protein that acts as the primary building base of all tissues within the body. Therefore, it is essential to healing wounds, the creation of new skin/scar tissue, and the list goes on.

The majority of us consume too many protein-rich foods in our daily lives. However, due to the fatigue and lack of appetite that surgery can cause, it is recommended to eat protein-rich foods to ensure that you get the nutrition that you require.

You can get protein from the following sources:

- Peanut butter sandwich
- Tuna salad
- Chicken Salad
- Refried beans
- Chocolate milk
- Meat soup

## Important tips to relax your throat while eating

The following tips listed below will be helpful while eating.

1. Drink water or any other fluid like soft drinks and juices while eating.
2. Add soups to your diet that will be easy to digest and don't cause acidity. Some of the recipes are listed in Chapter 6.
3. Eat slowly and chew the food properly so that it can easily be swallowed.
4. Incorporating cheese into stews and soups, mixing butter and milk, blending vegetables, adding beans and lentils in soups, eating them with dips such as hummus or sour cream, or making whey protein or the morning beverage mix in milkshakes are just a few ways to boost calories.

# Week 2: 7-day Meal Plan

|  | Breakfast | Lunch | Dinner | Snack |
|---|---|---|---|---|
| Day 1 | Scrambled Eggs with a chocolate smoothie<br><br>*Start your day with soft food | Chicken Breast Delight or Tuna Salad<br><br>*Tuna is a rich source of iodine | Vegetable stew with some gravy | Brazil nuts |
| Day 2 | Gluten-free toast and eggs | Vegetable Broth or Tahini Salmon | Angel Hair Pasta with Shrimp, Zucchini, and Pesto<br><br>*Use gluten-free pasta (it doesn't have to be angel hair). Iodine is abundant in shrimp. | 1 banana |
| Day 3 | Green Monster smoothie | Broccoli Soup with Turmeric and Ginger | Salmon and Asparagus | Brazil nuts |
| Day 4 | Yogurt with meshed dates | Asian-Style Vegetable Soup | Refried beans | Simple banana bread |
| Day 5 | Mashed Potatoes | Minestrone soup or vegetable | Steak with Olive Oil | Cashew butter green |

|  |  |  | stew |  | smoothie |
|---|---|---|---|---|---|
| Day 6 | Peanut butter sandwich | Lentil Soup or sweet potato soup | Chicken breast delight with garlic | Banana with flavored yogurt |
| Day 7 | Oatmeal | Spinach and Watercress Salad | Meat Soup | Honey roasted chickpeas |

# Sample Recipes

# Asian-Style Vegetable Soup

**Ingredients:**

- 1/3 large head of cabbage, shredded
- 1 medium or large head of bok choy, stem and leaves separated
- 9 artichoke hearts, drained
- 2 cups beef or venison, boiled and cubed
- 6 cups beef broth, preferably homemade
- 4 cups leafy green vegetables, chopped
- 1/3 lb. fresh or frozen broccoli, chopped
- 2 large organic carrots, sliced or diced
- 5 oz. water chestnuts, drained and diced or sliced
- 2 medium onions, sliced or diced
- 4 cloves garlic, minced
- 1/2-in. to 3-in. fresh ginger root, grated
- 2-4 tbsp. fat
- 1-1/2 tsp. rock salt or kosher salt
- ground black pepper, to taste
- 1 cup cauliflower, chopped

**Instructions:**

1. Melt your preferred fat using medium heat in a pot.
2. Sauté the onions for at least 5 minutes.
3. Stir in bok choy stems.
4. Continue stirring until onions and bok choy are translucent.

5. Add the garlic, carrots, cabbage, and ginger.
6. Stir around for 1 to 2 minutes.
7. Add the bok choy leaves and any other leafy green vegetables
8. Stir and cover for about a minute.
9. Pour in the beef broth.
10. Increase the heat to high.
11. Add the salt, pepper, artichokes, and meat.
12. Cover the pot with its lid.
13. Add the broccoli, cauliflower, and water chestnuts.
14. When the broth comes to a boil, reduce the heat to medium-low.
15. Cook for 5 to 15 minutes.
16. Serve hot with a side of soy sauce or grated cheese.

# Lentil Soup

**Ingredients:**

- 1 tbsp. avocado oil
- 1 cup onion, diced
- 1/2 cup carrot, diced
- 1/2 cup celery, diced
- 4 cups vegetable or chicken broth
- 1 cup dried red lentils, well rinsed
- 1/4 tsp dried thyme
- 1/2 cup fresh flat-leaf parsley, chopped
- salt and pepper, to taste

**Instructions:**

1. Sauté carrot, celery, and onion in a large saucepan over medium heat. Do so until they are soft.
2. Pour in the broth with lentils and thyme and wait to boil.
3. Lower the heat. Cover and leave to simmer until lentils are soft, about 20 minutes.
4. Transfer the soup into a blender.
5. Set the blender on high. Purée the soup until it's creamy.
6. If it's too thick, pour in a cup of water.
7. Add salt and pepper to taste.

8. Return to the saucepan to reheat if necessary.
9. Ladle into bowls and garnish with parsley.
10. Serve and enjoy while hot.

# Meaty Cauliflower Soup

**Ingredients:**

- 1 cup cauliflower, chopped
- 1/8 tsp. pepper
- 1/8 tsp. ground mustard
- 1 chicken stock
- 2-1/2 cups hot water
- fresh parsley, chopped

**Instructions:**

1. Heat a saucepan. Pour in water and condensed chicken broth.
2. Add cauliflower, mustard, and pepper.
3. Stir from time to time.
4. Adjust heat to high. Let it boil.
5. Reduce the heat. Allow it to simmer while covered.
6. Stir from time to time until potatoes are soft.
7. Add ham and add in half and half.
8. Cook for 5 more minutes, uncovered. Do not boil.
9. Turn off the heat as soon as the soup starts to simmer.
10. Top with parsley upon serving.

# Tomato and Basil Soup

## Ingredients:

- 1 medium-sized onion, chopped
- 1 clove garlic, sliced finely
- 2 tablespoons olive oil
- 3 pcs. vine tomatoes or 8 pcs. cherry tomatoes, chopped
- 400 g can plum tomatoes
- 150 ml water
- 5 leaves of fresh basil or 1 tsp. dried basil
- 1 tsp. salt
- pepper

## Instructions:

1. Sauté onion, tomatoes, garlic, and basil in olive oil.
2. Pour in the canned tomatoes. Add salt and pepper.
3. Cover and let it simmer for 30 minutes on low heat.
4. Transfer to a blender or food processor and blend until smooth.
5. Serve and enjoy.

# Sweet Potato Soup

**Ingredients:**

- 1 fennel bulb, chopped
- 1 fresh ginger, chopped into an inch
- 1 red onion, chopped
- 1 small fresh turmeric root, chopped
- 10 oz. frozen sweet potato cubes
- 12 oz. frozen cauliflower florets
- 2 cloves garlic, chopped
- black pepper
- sea salt
- fresh herbs, chopped
- water or 4 cups of veggie broth

**Instructions:**

1. Use a stovetop soup pot to combine all ingredients.
2. Boil the ingredients and simmer for 30 minutes until vegetables are tender and flavors have soaked into the broth.
3. Transfer the ingredients, by batch, into a blender. To achieve a chunkier soup, pulse a few times or blend to purée.
4. Top with fresh green herbs when served.

# Minestrone Soup

**Ingredients:**

- 3 large carrots, diced
- 2 large onions, chopped
- 2 cloves garlic, minced
- 2 cups celery, chopped
- 1 cup green beans, cut into half-inch pieces
- 1.5 cups kidney beans, dried
- 1 large bell pepper, diced
- 1 cup frozen peas
- 1 can tomatoes, diced
- 2 cups tomato sauce
- 2 tbsp. Fresh basil or 1 tsp. dried basil
- 6 cups water

**Instructions:**

1. In a stockpot over medium heat, add the water, onions, carrots, and celery.
2. As the water starts to bubble, add in the green beans, bell pepper, peas, and tomatoes.
3. Let it bubble for around 30 minutes.
4. Add water if necessary. The soup should be thick, similar to a stew, but not too thick.

5. After half an hour, add the tomato sauce, beans, basil, and salt to taste.
6. Let it stew for 5-10 additional minutes; at that point, include the garlic. Let it stew for 5 additional minutes.
7. Serve while hot.

# Broccoli Soup with Tumeric and Ginger

**Ingredients:**

- 1 onion
- 3 cloves garlic
- 1 can of unsweetened coconut milk
- 1 tsp. salt
- 1 tsp. turmeric powder
- 2 tsp. fresh ginger chopped
- 2 small heads of broccoli chopped into florets
- 1 cup of water
- Optional, for serving: fresh greens, roasted almonds, sesame seeds, and/or yogurt

**Instructions:**

1. In a pan over low heat, pour half of the coconut milk.
2. Add the garlic and onion. Cook until soft, for about 5 minutes.
3. Add the ginger, turmeric, florets, salt, water, and the rest of the coconut milk.
4. Simmer for an hour. Stir occasionally and mash the broccoli.
5. Allow the mixture to cool.
6. Blend the mixture in a food processor. Do it in batches if needed.
7. Serve with a choice of sides or toppings.

# Vegetable Stew

**Ingredients:**

- 3 tbsp. avocado oil, divided
- 1 cup parsley root, scraped and sliced thinly
- 1 cup mushrooms, cut in half if too big
- 4 leeks, sliced and green parts trimmed
- 1 cup russet potatoes, peeled and diced
- 1/4 tsp. thyme
- 2 bay leaves
- 2 turnips, peeled and cut into half-inch dice
- 2-1/2 cups apple cider vinegar
- 3 tbsp. Worcestershire sauce
- rosemary
- 1/2 lb. small Brussels sprouts, washed and trimmed
- 3 tbsp. flour
- 2 cups hot vegetable broth
- 3 tbsp. molasses
- 3 tsp. paprika
- salt
- pepper

**Instructions:**

1. Pour oil into a large, heavy pot.
2. Sauté the leeks, parsley roots, thyme, bay leaves, and rosemary until the leeks begin to turn golden.

3. Add the mushrooms and turnips to the pot, as well as the wine and the Worcestershire sauce. Stir and lower the flame.
4. Add them to the stew, stir again, and cover.
5. In a small, heavy saucepan, pour the remaining oil.
6. Cook the roux for a few minutes, then add the hot vegetable broth and stir quickly with a whisk.
7. Add the vinegar, molasses, and paprika. Whisk until the sauce is smooth and pour it over the stew.
8. Simmer the stew gently, covered, for an hour, or until all the vegetables are tender.
9. Season to taste with salt and pepper.
10. Serve hot.

# Garlic Hummus

**Ingredients:**

- 12 heads of garlic, roasted
- 2 tsp. virgin coconut oil
- 2 12-cup muffin tins
- extra trays of ice cube

**Instructions:**

1. Preheat the oven to 400°F.
2. Cut off the top of each garlic head to make the top of the cloves visible.
3. Put each garlic head in a muffin tin cup.
4. Rub the top of the garlic heads with coconut oil.
5. Use the second muffin tin to cover the first one.
6. Put in the oven and wait for 30 minutes to bake.
7. Take the garlic cloves out of the heads.
8. You may place 4-5 cloves of garlic in each ice cube tray section to store leftovers.
9. Use olive oil to cover cloves and freeze.
10. Squeeze the frozen roasted garlic cubes out of the trays and store them using a container.

# Salmon and Asparagus

**Ingredients:**

- 2 salmon filets
- 14-oz. young potatoes
- 8 asparagus spears, trimmed and halved
- 2 handfuls cherry tomatoes
- 1 handful basil leaves
- 2 tbsp. extra-virgin olive oil
- 1 tbsp. balsamic vinegar

**Instructions:**

1. Heat oven to 428°F.
2. Arrange potatoes into a baking dish.
3. Drizzle potatoes with extra-virgin olive oil.
4. Roast potatoes until they have turned golden brown.
5. Place asparagus into the baking dish together with the potatoes.
6. Roast in the oven for 15 minutes.
7. Arrange cherry tomatoes and salmon among the vegetables.
8. Drizzle with balsamic vinegar and the remaining olive oil.
9. Roast until the salmon is cooked.
10. Throw in basil leaves before transferring everything to a serving dish.
11. Serve while hot.

# Tahini Salmon

## Instructions:

- 1/4 cup tahini
- 3 tbsp. fresh lemon juice
- 1 tsp. mashed garlic
- 1/4 tsp. salt
- 1/2 cup finely chopped cilantro
- 2 tbsp. roughly chopped toasted walnuts
- 2 tbsp. roughly chopped toasted almonds
- 1 tbsp. finely chopped onion
- 1 tsp. extra-virgin olive oil
- cayenne
- black pepper, freshly ground
- 1 lb. wild salmon skin removed, fresh or frozen

## Instructions:

1. In a bowl, combine the tahini, 2 tbsp. of lemon juice, 3 tbsp. of water, mashed garlic, and 1/8 tsp. of salt; set aside
2. In a separate bowl, combine the cilantro, walnuts, almonds, onion, olive oil, cayenne, black pepper, and 1/8 tsp. of salt.
3. Fill the bottom of a steamer with water and bring to a boil.
4. Season fish with 1 tbsp. of lemon juice.

5. Place it on a plate and put it on top of the steamer. Cover and cook, taking care to remove while the fish is still pink inside, about 3 to 4 minutes.
6. Remove the fish from the steamer, top with the tahini mixture, and then with the cilantro mixture.
7. Serve warm or at room temperature.

# Chicken Breast Delight

**Ingredients:**

- 1 tsp. dried oregano
- 1/2 tsp. rosemary
- 1/2 tsp. garlic powder
- 1/8 tsp. salt
- finely ground black pepper
- 4 chicken breasts

**Instructions:**

1. Remove any fat from the breasts.
2. Mix the remaining ingredients in a separate container.
3. Add the mixture on either side of the chicken.
4. Prepare a frying pan, lightly oil the pan, and set the stove to medium.
5. Add the chicken to the frying pan. Cook for 3 to 5 minutes on each face.
6. Cool the chicken for a couple of minutes after cooking.
7. Serve warm.

# Steak with Olive Oil

## Ingredients:

- 2 8-oz. grass-fed New York strip steaks, about 1-1/2-inch-thick, trimmed
- 3 tbsp. olive oil, divided
- 1 tsp. freshly ground black pepper, divided
- 1 tsp. kosher salt, divided
- 1 garlic clove, crushed
- 1 rosemary sprig
- optional: rosemary leaves

## Instructions:

1. Place the grill pan over medium-high heat.
2. Brush a tablespoon of oil on the steak, then sprinkle with half a teaspoon of salt and another half teaspoon of pepper.
3. Put a tablespoon of oil into the pan, followed by a rosemary sprig and garlic.
4. Cook steak for about 9 minutes, or until preferred doneness is achieved. For every minute, turn the steak and baste it with oil.
5. Transfer the steak to a cutting board, letting it rest for 5 minutes.

6. Slice steak across the grain and place on a platter. Drizzle with the juice from the cutting board and the leftover oil.
7. Sprinkle it with the remaining salt and pepper.
8. Upon serving, garnish with rosemary leaves, if desired.

# Garlic Broccoli Salad

## Ingredients:

- 1 head broccoli, cut into florets
- 1 tsp. olive oil
- 1-1/2 tbsp. rice wine vinegar
- 1 tbsp. sesame oil
- 2 cloves garlic, minced
- 1 pinch of cayenne pepper
- 3 tbsp. golden raisins

## Instructions:

1. Fill water into a steamer. Bring to a boil.
2. Add broccoli. Cover. Steam until tender for about 3 minutes.
3. Rinse broccoli and set aside.
4. Heat olive oil in a skillet over medium heat.
5. Put in pine nuts. Stir fry for 1-2 minutes.
6. Remove from heat.
7. Whisk together rice vinegar, sesame oil, pepper, and garlic.
8. Transfer the broccoli, nuts, and raisins to the rice vinegar dressing.
9. Serve and enjoy.

# Spinach and Watercress Salad

**Ingredients:**

- 1 cup watercress, washed with stems removed
- 3 cups baby spinach, washed with stems removed
- 1 medium sliced avocado
- 1/4 cup avocado oil
- 1/8 cup lemon juice
- a pinch of salt

**Instructions:**

1. Pat dry the spinach and watercress. Remove the stem and separate the leaves.
2. On a large serving plate, combine the leaves of the watercress and the spinach.
3. Cut the avocado in half, then remove the pit. Peel the skin off from each side.
4. Slice the avocados into thin strips. Set aside.
5. Prepare the dressing by combining avocado oil and lemon juice.
6. Arrange the avocado strips on top of the watercress and spinach.
7. Season with salt and pepper.

## Vegetable Broth

**Ingredients:**

- 1 tbsp. oil
- 2 leeks, sliced
- 2 carrots, sliced
- 2 ribs celery
- 1/4 tsp. salt
- 8 cups water

To make the soup:

- 1 tbsp. oil
- 2 cups potatoes, diced
- 1 cup mushrooms, diced
- 1-1/2 cups cauliflower, diced
- 1 cup onion, diced
- 1 cup celery, diced
- 1 cup carrot, diced
- 1-1/2 cups red beans, cooked
- 2 sprigs rosemary
- 4 sprigs thyme
- 2 cups spinach

**Instructions:**

1. To a pot on medium heat, add oil and leeks.
2. Cook for about three minutes or until they start to soften up.

3. Add carrots and top of a few celery stalks with leaves.
4. Cover with water.
5. Add salt. Bring to a simmer and cook until carrots are tender but not mushy.
6. Turn off the heat and let it cool down a little.
7. When the broth has cooled down, strain out the veggies.
8. Remove carrots and set them aside.
9. Squeeze most of the liquid out of the leeks and celery.

To cook the soup:

1. Add carrots to some of the broth and blend.
2. Add oil, onions, raw carrots, and celery in a pot on medium heat. Cook until onions are translucent, approximately 3 to 5 minutes.
3. Add broth, potatoes, and herbs.
4. Bring to a simmer and cook for 10 minutes.
5. Add cauliflower and red beans.
6. Simmer for another 5 minutes.
7. Add the package of frozen green beans and cook until the potatoes and cauliflower are tender, approximately for another 5 minutes.
8. At the end of cooking, add spinach.
9. Serve warm.

# Fruit and Dark Greens Salad

**Ingredients:**

- 1 cup watermelon
- 1 cup cucumber sliced or spiral
- 1/2 cup raspberries
- 1 sliced avocado
- 1 cup baby broccoli
- 1 cup papaya
- 1/2 cup toasted almonds
- 4 cups baby kale

Dressing:

- 1/2 cup olive oil
- 1/2 cup master tonic
- 1/4 cup goji berries
- 4 dates
- a pinch of sea salt

Tonic:

- 1/4 cup garlic, minced
- 1/4 cup onion, chopped
- 2 tbsp. horseradish, minced
- 2 knobs of turmeric, chopped
- 1 jalapeno pepper, chopped
- 32 oz. organic apple cider vinegar
- 1/4 cup fresh ginger, chopped

- juice of 1 lemon

**Instructions:**

1. Mix all salad ingredients except almonds.
2. Toss salad.

To make the dressing:

1. Mix the master tonic, olive oil, and salt.
2. In a blender, blend goji berries and dates until smooth.
3. Upon serving the salad, drizzle the dressing on, and gently add almonds.

To make the master tonic:

1. Add all ingredients to apple cider vinegar.
2. Blend all ingredients until everything is mixed well.
3. Let tonic sit in a jar for 1 to 2 weeks, shaking periodically.
4. Strain first before adding the leftover vinegar mixture into a jar with a cover.

# Conclusion

Congratulations on concluding our comprehensive guide on the thyroidectomy procedure and the post-thyroidectomy diet. By now, you should have a well-rounded understanding of what a thyroidectomy entails and the steps you can take to ensure a smooth recovery through proper nutrition. You've taken an important step in prioritizing your health and well-being, and for that, you deserve heartfelt applause.

You've learned about the different types of thyroidectomy procedures and the reasons one might undergo such surgery. Whether it's due to cancer, hyperthyroidism, or another condition affecting the gland, the decision to proceed with a thyroidectomy is significant and often comes after much consideration and consultation with health professionals.

As you embark on the journey of recovery, remember that patience and self-care are your allies. The post-surgical period may present its challenges, but armed with knowledge and a supportive medical team, you are more than capable of navigating this path. Adjustments won't happen overnight, and it's perfectly normal to experience a range of emotions as you adapt to your new normal.

The role of diet in your recovery has been a central theme of this guide. You now understand the importance of maintaining a balanced intake of nutrients to support healing and facilitate the management of your thyroid hormone levels. By focusing on foods rich in calcium and iodine and staying hydrated, you are giving your body the building blocks it needs to recuperate and function optimally.

You've also learned how to mindfully approach dietary changes, listen to your body's cues, and work closely with a registered dietitian. It's vital to understand that everyone's path to recovery is individual, and a method that benefits one person may not be the most suitable for another. Therefore, personalization and flexibility in your diet plan are key.

Let's not forget the significance of regular follow-up appointments with your healthcare provider. Monitoring your progress and making necessary adjustments to your medication and diet are essential steps to ensure your continued health and well-being. Take pride in every small victory along the way—each one is a testament to your resilience and commitment to taking control of your health.

In the spirit of encouragement, I urge you to look ahead with optimism. Remember, a thyroidectomy is not merely an end but a new beginning. It marks the start of a journey toward renewed health, and with the right care, you have the potential to lead a full and active life.

I want to take this moment to thank you sincerely for trusting this guide as a resource in your post-thyroidectomy journey. Your dedication to reading through the information provided and your proactive stance in managing your health is commendable. Your perseverance and positive mindset are what will carry you forward into a future of wellness and vitality.

As you move forward, continue to embrace the support of friends, family, and fellow patients who understand what you're going through. There is a strong community out there, ready to share their experiences and offer advice. Do not hesitate to reach out and connect; the shared wisdom and encouragement can be incredibly uplifting.

To wrap up, remember that a successful recovery is a collaborative effort between you, your healthcare team, and your loved ones. Stay informed, stay nourished, and stay hopeful. A thyroidectomy may have been a necessary step for your health, but it does not define who you are. You are a person of strength and resilience, capable of overcoming obstacles and emerging stronger on the other side.

Thank you once again for completing this guide. We wish you the very best in your continued journey toward health and happiness. Here's to a bright and thriving future!

# FAQ

**What is a thyroidectomy and when is it necessary?**

A thyroidectomy is a surgical procedure to remove all or part of the thyroid gland. It's commonly performed for conditions such as thyroid cancer, large goiters, overactive thyroid (hyperthyroidism), or non-cancerous enlargement of the thyroid (benign nodules) that may cause difficulty in breathing or swallowing.

**How should I prepare for a thyroidectomy?**

Preparation for a thyroidectomy typically involves several pre-surgical evaluations, including blood tests, imaging studies, and possibly a fine needle aspiration biopsy if cancer is suspected. Your doctor may also instruct you on medication adjustments and fasting requirements before surgery. It is important to follow all pre-operative instructions to ensure your safety and the success of the procedure.

### What can I expect during the recovery period after a thyroidectomy?

Post-thyroidectomy, you may experience pain at the incision site, hoarseness, or temporary changes in your voice. Your doctor will prescribe medications for pain management and any necessary hormone replacements. Recovery varies from person to person, but most individuals can resume normal activities within a few weeks, following their doctor's guidance.

### Will I need to take medication after my thyroid has been removed?

Yes, if your entire thyroid is removed, you will need to take thyroid hormone replacement medication for life to substitute for the hormones no longer being produced naturally. Your doctor will monitor your hormone levels regularly to adjust your dosage as needed.

### How long after a thyroidectomy can I start the post-thyroidectomy diet?

You can usually start the post-thyroidectomy diet as soon as you feel comfortable swallowing after the surgery. This could be as soon as the same day or the day after. Start with liquids and soft foods, then gradually introduce more solid foods as tolerated. Always follow your surgeon's specific dietary recommendations.

## Are there any foods I should avoid following a thyroidectomy?

Immediately following surgery, you might need to avoid foods that are hard to chew or swallow. In the long term, depending on whether you need to take calcium or iodine supplements, certain foods high in these minerals might need to be moderated. These specifics should be discussed with your healthcare professional based on your individual needs.

## How does diet impact my recovery and overall health after a thyroidectomy?

Diet plays a crucial role in your recovery and ongoing health after a thyroidectomy. Consuming a balanced diet rich in fruits, vegetables, lean proteins, and whole grains can help promote healing and manage your energy levels. Adequate intake of specific nutrients like calcium and vitamin D is important, especially if your parathyroid glands were affected during surgery, which can impact calcium metabolism. Your healthcare provider or a registered dietitian can give you personalized advice for your diet post-thyroidectomy.

# References and Helpful Links

J. L. D. N. (2023, September 21). 14-Day Meal Plan For Hypothyroidism And Weight Loss | Diet vs Disease. Diet Vs Disease. https://www.dietvsdisease.org/meal-plan-for-hypothyroidism-and-weight-loss/

Cdn, N. R. M. R. (2020, August 20). 8 fantastic foods to boost your body's Vitamin D (Plus recipes!). Healthline. https://www.healthline.com/health/nutrition/vitamin-d-foods

Berkheiser, K. (2023, February 1). 9 Healthy foods that are rich in iodine. Healthline. https://www.healthline.com/nutrition/iodine-rich-foods#:~:text=The%20Bottom%20Line&text=The%20foods%20highest%20in%20iodine,add%20iodine%20to%20your%20meals.

Healthdirect Australia. (n.d.). Total thyroidectomy (for thyrotoxicosis). Healthdirect. https://www.healthdirect.gov.au/surgery/total-thyroidectomy-for-thyrotoxicosis

(Thyroidectomy Diet, n.d.)

Koeplin, M., MD. (2018, June 12). Eating & Your Diet after LINX surgery | Dr. Michael Koeplin, MD. Dr. Michael Koeplin. https://michaelkoeplinmd.com/eating-your-diet-after-linx-surgery/

Professional, C. C. M. (n.d.). Graves' disease. Cleveland Clinic. https://my.clevelandclinic.org/health/diseases/15244-graves-disease

Professional, C. C. M. (n.d.-b). Hashimoto's Disease. Cleveland Clinic. https://my.clevelandclinic.org/health/diseases/17665-hashimotos-disease

Professional, C. C. M. (n.d.-c). Postpartum thyroiditis. Cleveland Clinic. https://my.clevelandclinic.org/health/diseases/15294-postpartum-thyroiditis

Rd, K. M. M. (2022, February 22). 5 tips for what to eat after thyroid surgery. Low Iodine Dietitian. https://lowiodinedietitian.com/what_to_eat_after_thyroid_surgery/

Thyroid gland | You and Your Hormones from the Society for Endocrinology. (n.d.). https://www.yourhormones.info/glands/thyroid-gland/

Stang, D. (2019, October 31). Thyroid gland removal. Healthline. https://www.healthline.com/health/thyroid-gland-removal

Thyroid lobectomy: removal of half of thyroid. (n.d.). https://www.thyroidcancer.com/thyroid-cancer-surgery/thyroid-lobectomy

Professional, C. C. M. (n.d.-d). Thyroid nodules. Cleveland Clinic. https://my.clevelandclinic.org/health/diseases/13121-thyroid-nodule

Thyroidectomy. (n.d.). Cleveland Clinic. Retrieved August 25, 2022, from https://my.clevelandclinic.org/health/treatments/7016-thyroidectomy.

Professional, C. C. M. (n.d.-e). Thyroiditis. Cleveland Clinic. https://my.clevelandclinic.org/health/diseases/15455-thyroiditis

Made in the USA
Coppell, TX
14 January 2025